Outsmarting the **Dementia** Epidemic:

7 Key Memory Care Actions
To Avoid Alzheimer's and
Successfully Keep Your Brain
Safe, Sharp and Sexy
Into the Future

DEDICATION

To all of those who have come before me struggling with memory and other cognitive functions. And to those dedicated professionals and family members caregivers who are devoted to caring for those with Alzheimer's and dementia. May this book be able to fulfill my mission of preventing a million cases of Alzheimer's. My intention is to alert the person on the street --whether reading this book, watching news talk shows, seeing movies, or watching online educational videos -- as to how they might be able to avoid a future of "forgetting who they are, where they are, and who their loved ones are" because of avoidable brain degeneration.

Outsmarting the **Dementia** Epidemic

7 Key Memory Care Actions To Avoid Alzheimer's and Successfully Keep Your Brain Safe, Sharp and Sexy Into the Future

Dr. Jay Sordean

Best-Selling Author & Clinician

Appearing on

ABC, CBS, NBC, FOX, and CW

CONTENTS

THANKS AND ACKNOWLEDGEMENTS

The input, ideas, and support of many people made this book a reality. My thanks go out to those here now and those whose influence in the past continues with me today. Including:

My Family Members, John Sordean, Hattie Sordean, Uncle Russ Lamb, Aunt Judy Lamb, Aunt Dottie Sordean, Andrea Mintzer, Judy Sordean, Eliot Mintzer, Sigal Gafni, Savyon Gafni Sordean, Elah Gafni Sordean, Cathy Frakes, Donna Geniti, Erelah Gafni, Layla Gafni Kubukeli, Randy Lamb, Priscilla Johnson, other family members on the Sordean, Bridgford, Lamb and Gafni lineages, including cousins, nieces, nephews, and once-removeds and grand- and great-grandparents.

Interviewees: Byron Fong LAc, Austin Hill Shaw, Joanny Liu OMD, Geoff Olsen, Joseph Smith DC, Michael Nelson MD, Rob DeMartino DC, Kewesi Simon, Deborah Rozman PhD, Ben Bernstein PhD, Doug Kempton DC, Renee Dyer, Katinka Van dermerwe DC, Don Lawson, Cori Stern DC, Belinda Leung, Michael Gelbart PhD, Erica Shaver-Nelson, Marsha Peoples, Anne Sanabria, Shirley McElhatten, Micheal Pope PhD, David Blyweiss MD, Sergio Azzolino DC.

Other Resources: Aristo Vodjani PhD, Jeffrey S. Bland PhD, Colette Jones, Rick Huntoon DC, Marshal Mermel, Simon Gibson PT, Jon Mazura MD, Pam Grant-Ryan.

People I have studied with or learned from in various ways: Michael E. Lara, MD, Paul Witcomb DC, Datis Kharrazian DC, Martin Katz, Jared Kneebone, Michael Pearce DC, Dr. Dale Bredesen, Tony Robbins, John Assaraf, Benjamin Levy, Blair Singer, Richard Bandler, John Grinder, A.M. Krasner, Father Richard Mapplebeckpalmer, Frank Lamport, George Rodkey, Thom Hartmann, Mark Yuzuik, Simone Coulars, Joel Roberts, Roger Love, Cheri Tree, Lao Tzu, Chuang Tzu, The Dailai Lama, Miki Shima OMD, Matt VanBenschoten OMD, and many others.

TV affiliates: Clint Arthur and Alison Savitch, Adrienne Williams, Jennifer Schack, Izzy Karpinski, Alex Maragos, Adina Klein, Cory McPherrin, Kara Sewell, Jemelle Holopirek, Amanda Sanchez, Taylor Tucker, Raynard Gadson, Kristina Behr, JD Roberto, Cynthia Newell, Celina Tuason, Monica Jackson, Victoria Spilabotte, Tiffany Frowiss, Renee Kohn, Susan Hancock, John Carter, Holly Hendrick, Leslie Williams, Tom Crawford, Oprah, Mark Harmon.

Thousands of patients I have had the pleasure and honor to work with over the last 30+ years.

Friends and Acquaintances world-wide. And everyone who bought (and hopefully read) this book and made it a bestseller.

Hand-drawn pictures by Simone Coulars. All other pictures and charts by Jay Sordean, rights obtained, or credited as noted.

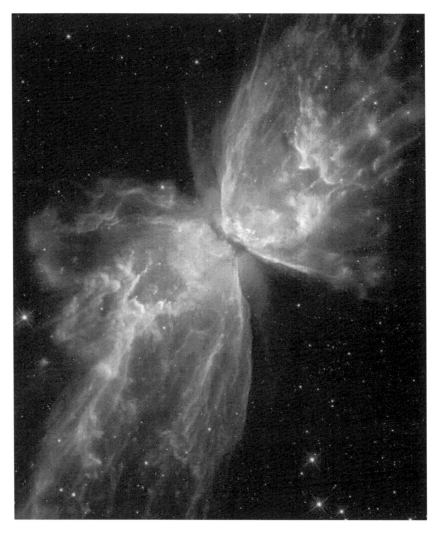

Scientists tell us:

There are 100 billion galaxies in our Universe

There are 100 billion stars in our Galaxy (The Milky Way)

The Earth is 4.4 billion years old

There are 50 billion cells in your brain &

There are 1,000 trillion synapses (connections) between your brain cells.

INTRODUCTION: Your Brain is Shouting "FORGET ME, NOT!"

As you sit here reading this sentence, your brain is talking to you. Shortly, as your brain reads these words your brain will (now) tell you that there is a chance that it, and thus you, will suffer early brain death at the hands of dementia and Alzheimer's. This is whether you have a family history of Alzheimer's or other forms of dementia - or not. One in eight Americans have Alzheimer's and one in three Americans dies with some form of dementia.

Obviously, when we think about it, our individual brains do not operation in isolation. Our brains, like the Internet, are connected to little servers. What are these little servers? Storing memories, information, analytical skills, emotional content, and language communication experiences? When we talk to each other, when we read a book, when we do research, all of these activities are mediated through our own brain and the complex interactions between different brains. And thus, in reality, when our memory is functioning, it is a pass-through function of the brain. So in fact, if we have fears -- based on likelihood or family experience of early brain death, in other words dementia and Alzheimer's -- these fears are mediated as a function of our brain, the cerebral cortex, and survival brainstem. In fact, the title of this chapter, "Forget me, NOT!" is your brain calling out for the rest of you, in conjunction and cooperation with the brain, to take action and do everything possible for the survival and thriving of your brain. (Which incidentally means that you have to take care of others too because they are servers in your network.)

The Dementia Epidemic and Plague

Why do I call this the "'plague' of early brain death syndrome and

Alzheimer's?" It is a plague and epidemic because it is so prevalent and expanding. It is also a condition that causes great consternation, emotional distress and challenges to the caregivers around you, whether they be children, grandchildren, spouses or paid professionals.

The major cause of bankruptcy in the United States is medical and healthcare costs. If you don't know already, people with moderate and advanced Alzheimer's have to be taken care of constantly as if they were infants. This exacts not only a huge financial toll but also an emotional toll. As you think about these possibilities, your brain is no doubt saying, "Take care of me. I don't want to end up that way. I want to stay healthy, alive, vibrant, engaged, active, thinking and feeling and communicating with others up until the day the entire body decides to give out and take its last breath and heart beat."

So, do your brain a favor and take action now. Read this -- follow the 7 Key Memory Care Actions of this program to increase the odds of having a lasting, enduring, and glowing memory into the future. No matter how old or young you are, it is never too early to start.

Let me convince you again to "Forget me NOT" and to help me in my mission to prevent a million "cases" of Alzheimer's and dementia.

Key Memory Care Actions

As the bestselling author of the new book, "Super Brain: Maximize Your Brain Health for a Better Life," I have discovered a number of medically sound, key factors that can either help you enhance your brain health and function or set it up for early failure. We all want to enhance our brain health and function, don't we? At the same time we should pay attention to factors that will set our brain up for failure. After all, arguably, your brain is your greatest asset.

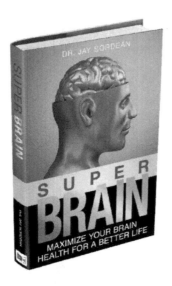

Number 1 Bestselling Book that Complements This One

Improving brain function has unbelievably valuable benefits. On the other hand, brain degeneration and dementia have devastatingly damaging impact on our own lives and on those around us. Choose wisely. Either you work to help your brain or you damage it.

It is "Maintain-Your-Brain Time!"

Are you feeling forgetful? Well, NOW is "maintain-your-brain" time. It's rarely too late, and never too early to start thinking about protecting your memory and other important brain functions. Your brain has a remarkable ability to adapt and change to help maintain and repair important communication functions in the body. This changeability is called "neuroplasticity." Your neuroplasticity is greatly aided by eating a healthy diet and making other positive lifestyle changes—including quitting smoking, losing weight, exercise, and sufficient sleep.

Keeping your body in good working order—like controlling blood sugar levels and reducing chronic inflammation and stress—also keeps the brain and entire nervous system functioning in a much healthier manner.

So, in addition to the content of this book, we also offer you other important resources at the end of each chapter and at the end of this book.

RESOURCES

When you purchase a hard copy of this book as well as this e-book, send a copy of your receipts to outsmartingdementia@gmail.com and we will send you a pdf version of this e-book. You will also be eligible to receive the analysis of a brief online survey of your basic brain health when you complete the online survey. We will send you a link for this brain survey after we receive your receipt.

Purchase of this book and "SUPER BRAIN: Maximize Your Brain Health For a Better Life" entitles you to a 27% discount off of the comprehensive examination and evaluation of your health and nervous system at designated clinic locations within 4 months of purchase. The details of the different levels of evaluation and analysis will be emailed you after receipt of your book purchase invoices.

We also have a series of lectures / webinars you can subscribe to and that will be delivered to you to watch on your computer.

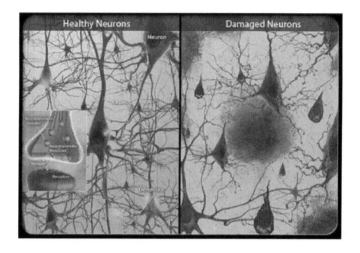

What can happen if you don't take care of your brain, nervous systems and body?

Picture of the tangles and debris in brains with damaged nerves compared to healthy nerves

CHAPTER 1   DEMENTIA, ALZHEIMER'S and WHAT BRAIN DEGENERATION LOOKS LIKE

DO YOU HAVE ANY OF THESE? WHAT DOES EARLY DEGENERATION OF THE BRAIN LOOK LIKE?

<u>The Primary Signs of Brain Degeneration include:</u>

Hypertension/High Blood Pressure

Poor Digestion

Allergies, food or otherwise*

Acid reflux*

Dry eyes and mouth*

Sexual Dysfunction

Erectile Dysfunction*

Hormone Imbalance

Increased Cholesterol*

Incontinence

Short-term Memory Issues

Memory Problems*

Reduced Ability to Learn

Mood Swings

Depression*

Lowered Attention Span

Fatigue

Lowered Creativity

Sleep problems*

Sleepiness when Reading

Reduced Comprehension

Inability to Handle Motion

(Like those crazy kids!)

Autoimmune disorders*

(Items marked with a * can also be observed with unequal brain development as well as brain degeneration)

Ask yourself honestly, do you recognize yourself in any of these? If you have recurring symptoms they can become permanent issues. So the symptoms that start out as annoyances can turn into more serious symptoms and issues that are very hard to turn around. If they can be turned around. This is just like a car with bad shock absorbers that will get worse and worse with time. The ride will become more and more uncomfortable. With teeth jarring shakes when hitting potholes. Well, like the evidence of the breaking down car, your bodily symptoms that go on and on point to chronicity.

What is it Like to Be a Person with Alzheimer's?

Coma and Alzheimer's - How They Compare

Do you ever wonder what is going inside the head and heart and mind of a person with moderate or advanced dementia? If you have ever worked with someone who has this condition, you'll begin to wonder why they behave as they do. In a slightly similar vein, if you have ever been around someone who is in a coma, well that person is obviously unable to move around very

8

much or to interact with the people around them. They are bedridden and can hardly move. People sitting next to someone in a coma can speak and talk to them but does the person in a coma hear them? People who have had the experience of coming out of a coma have said that they were able to actually hear voices but they cannot communicate back.

Alzheimer's, on the other hand, can be a situation in which a person is unable to speak, or is using a language known only to themselves. The individual can move around, can typically eat, and depending on the severity, is able to play games, able to follow some directions, occasionally go on field trips, do exercises and group-guided games, do art projects and listen to music.

In spite of this seeming to be functional in many ways, and getting up and moving around, the individual was severe Alzheimer's and dementia may actually be in a coma-like state internally. How could this be?

Have you ever driven a car for hours and hours on a long trip, perhaps listening to music, having an intense conversation with someone else, or being quiet and noticing the scenery go by? You have that ability to drive for hours and hours and hours on end and arriving at the destination going "Wow. That was really fast. I don't remember much of any of the driving." This is a clear indication of how we are able to operate on automatic pilot. Our breathing, our heart beating, and numerous other functions in the body operate automatically without our having to consciously think or remember to do so.

So the individual with Alzheimer's and dementia is able to do a number of tasks in this automatic fashion, unlike the person in a coma. Of course, the person in a coma may be able to breathe and the heart may work fine but they're not able to actually move their bodies and get their muscles to move. So all of this being said, it still leaves us with the question: "What is going on inside the brain, heart and mind of the person with Alzheimer's when they themselves cannot n I describe it very well or are unable to speak to us at all?" And even if they are speaking to us, is it a real, ongoing, awakened-state reality to them? Or is it a rote process where they are speaking and talking to us and from the outside it looks like normal but from the inside nothing is going on?

Certainly, the experts in the field state that working with the person with Alzheimer's keeps you "in the moment." Keeping present and focused in the now is a key to interacting with the Alzheimer's patient, even when you yourself may be thinking about future events and consequences. If you are at their level you are definitely in the moment and not thinking about the future or the past.

So, the above description may be what is going on inside the mind, head and heart of the personal with Alzheimer's. And even perhaps quite similar to the experience of an infant or toddler, except that they are taking in and remembering the experiences, or at least we assume as much even though they also do not have the verbal capability to express it in words.

My Experience of the "Alzheimer's Mind"?

I personally had this experience many years ago, having had an injury to one side of my head. For approximately four hours I experienced what I can only assume was an Alzheimer's-like experience. It was a complete blank for me in spite of my interacting with my wife Sigal, doctors and staff at the emergency room, and others. My interactions and "conversations" with others during those 4 hours are known to me only due to Sigal's telling me what happened – what I said, how she answered back, how I kept repeating the same questions over and over again with no apparent comprehension of what she was answering, how I answered the doctors questions (to see if I was oriented in time and space), and what was done in the ER itself.

The Beginning: I remember clearly looking into the mirror in our small apartment bathroom, seeing blood running out of a gash in my forehead. Sigal asked what happened and I said "maybe I was hit in the head by a so-called homeless person" or "maybe I hit my head on the metal security gate as I opened it to enter the apartment building" or "maybe I hit myself on some low hanging limb over the sidewalk" or even "maybe it was an alien abduction." Okay, well it was in Berkeley, California, and there had been a spate of people being mugged randomly with baseball bats. At the time of the blow to the head I think I had a list of 11 possible causes because I had no clear memory of what really happened.

This happened around 11 PM. Earlier Sigal had visited me in a coffee shop on Telegraph Avenue where I was reading a book called "The Tibetan

Book of Living and Dying." I remembered that just before I left the coffee shop I had finished a chapter that ended with the statement that, as humans, we have in common the reality that we never know when we will die. Ironic.

So during the interaction in the bathroom she said that maybe I had a concussion and that I should maybe lie down. I said "No, you shouldn't lie down with a concussion." That much I knew of my medical training. I also asked her, "Do we have medical insurance?" She said "Yes, but we have a high deductible." I said something like, "Oh that is not good. Do we have medical insurance?" And this apparently went on for some time, as her answer did not register in my brain and cause me to stop asking the question for at least 15 more rounds.

The Middle: We went to the Emergency Room at Alta Bates Hospital, about 10 minutes from the apartment. I knew the area very well and had also worked as a clerk in the Alta Bates Hospital ER in the mid 80's. Thus, I was the one to direct us by car to the ER although I have no recollection of that. I was functioning as the navigator but have no memory of having done so.

When we arrived in the ER, there was the usual intake triage, clean-up of the wound, the ER doctor sewing up my gash, the bandages applied, and the medications prescribed. At least I was told this is what happened and I could see the stitches later.

The End: What I do remember was suddenly waking up around 3 am or so in the waiting room of the ER. My eyes opened and I saw the clock on the wall. I looked at Sigal and asked "Do we have medical insurance?" She answered "Yes, but we have a high deductible." I didn't ask the question again, and she then knew that something had changed with me. As for me? It just seemed like I had been asleep and had some glimpses of an odd dream I had had.

Is it Really Like "Alzheimer's Mind"?

Can I say that this is what it is like for someone with significant dementia or Alzheimer's? No, but it did give me a glimpse at what it might be like given that my behaviors on the outside were similar to what one might see with someone with Alzheimer's or dementia. If it is similar, perhaps this might also be likened to sleep walking or walking around in a "movement-functional coma." People who sleep walk have told me that they did not remember what had occurred while they were out doing things around town in their pajamas. But those people woke up and were able to function fully the next day. People with significant dementia or Alzheimer's may be living a life that is something like sleep walking.

While we don't know for sure what is going on inside the head and life of someone with advanced dementia and Alzheimer's, we still can look at the symptoms and conditions we listed as related to them.   At first you might wonder what brain degeneration has to do with the list of symptoms or conditions. Many of them make sense, like short-term memory Issues, reduced ability to learn, lowered attention span, lowered creativity, sleepiness when reading, reduced comprehension, depression, fatigue and Inability to handle motion. These all make sense because they are easy to associate with brain function or lack thereof.

But what about the other things? Hypertension, Poor Digestion, Sexual Dysfunction, Hormone Imbalance, Incontinence, Mood Swings, Depression, and fatigue? Even if you are a cyber- hypochondriac, brain degeneration is not the first thing that comes to mind with these conditions, but indeed they could be a sign of brain degeneration as well as due to other physiological causes.

This is because your brain regulates all of the functions of your body, in conjunction with the endocrine (hormone) and immunological systems. Different types of dementia are associated with particular types of brain cell damage in particular regions of the brain. And these regions have different functions. To learn more about these functions, read <u>Super Brain: Maximize Your Brain Health for a Better Life.</u>

Please note also that the items in the list marked with an Asterisk * are also seen with an imbalanced development of the two hemispheres of the brain. Not only can that imbalance cause those symptoms but it could also help create the foundation for brain degeneration, like dementia and Alzheimer's, (not to mention ADD, ADHD, autism spectrum disorder, late speaking and other conditions of developmental dysfunction syndrome.) .

Now, Go Back to the List of Markers at the Top of (this) chapter

Again, it is worth repeating. The bottom ine question though becomes "Do you recognize yourself in any of these?" Recurring symptoms and conditions can become permanent issues. So the symptoms that start out as annoyances can turn into more serious symptoms and issues that are very hard to turn around. IF they can be turned around.

So, try to get healthy naturally. Your alternative is a chemical respirator of endless medication. And those medications don't work forever due to tolerance and declining efficacy. And what might these be?

As of 2015, The Food and Drug Administration (FDA) has approved two types of drugs specifically to treat symptoms of Alzheimer's disease, cholinesterase inhibitors and Memantine. The three approved cholinesterase inhibitors include the following:

•Donepezil (Aricept) is approved to treat all stages of Alzheimer's – can cause delirium

•Rivastigmine (Exelon) is approved to treat mild to moderate Alzheimer's.

•Galantamine (Razadyne) is approved to treat mild to moderate Alzheimer's.

They all lose effectiveness over time, just like recurring symptoms are an indication that the underlying cause is not changing and function continues to deteriorate.

Fill out this SURVEY of BRAIN HEALTH to see where you stand.

Enter the appropriate number - 0, 1, 2or 3 - with 0 as least/never and 3 as most/always

____Is your memory noticeably declining?

____Are you having a hard time remembering names and phone numbers?

____Is your ability to focus noticeably declining?

___Has it become harder for you to learn things?

___How often do you have a hard time remembering your appointments?

___Is your temperament getting worse in general?

___Are you losing your attention span endurance?

___How often do you find yourself down or sad?

___How often do you fatigue when driving compared to the past?

___How often do you walk into rooms and forget why?

___How often do you pick up your cell phone and forget why?

___TOTAL

If your total is 6 or more I suggest that you get evaluated more in depth. See Chapter 12

CHAPTER 2: TEN WARNING SIGNS OF ALZHEIMER'S

What are the 10 most important warning signs of the start of or progression of Alzheimer's? (According to the Alzheimer's Association)

1. Memory loss that disturbs daily life, especially forgetting recently learned information.

2. Challenges in planning or solving problems that they are familiar with.

3. Difficulty finishing familiar tasks at home or at work. Or at leisure.

4. Confusion with time and place. Similar to what happens with concussion.

5. Trouble understanding visual images and spacial relationships.

6. New problems with words in speaking and writing.

7. Misplacing things and losing the ability to retrace steps.

8. Decreased or poor judgments.

9. Withdrawal from work or social activities.

10. Changes in mood and personality. This can also be seen with concussions.

If you or your loved one has these signs, contact a competent physician or other medical professional who is experienced in assessing these conditions as misdiagnosis can occur. If an appointment takes t0o long to get, call the ER. This is how seriously you should take this.

You can get a copy of the 10 Warning Signs checklist created by the Alzheimer's Association for you to take to your physician by going to this link. http://www.TheRedwoodClinic.com/10signs

CHAPTER 3: THREE THINGS TO AVOID TO HELP PREVENT ALZHEIMER'S AND DEMENTIA

According to the Alzheimer's Association, Alzheimer's is one of 13 forms of dementia. Some others claim there are 80 forms of dementia. No matter what the actual number is, what is not disputed is that Alzheimer's is the most common type of dementia. The different types of dementia are distinguished by and based on symptoms and causes. Dementia in any form is something that you want to avoid if at all possible. A list of the types of dementia is shown later in this chapter.

I believe that the reason why you want to avoid memory loss and weakness is self-evident. Nevertheless, I find it surprising the responses I get from many people in the lectures I have given to community groups on the subject of how to take care of your brain and memory. Most of the people in the audience did not take the high risk of developing dementia seriously. I don't understand why this is the case. This is particularly disturbing to me because the majority of the audience members at my lectures have been 50 or older! Perhaps they listen to their doctors' dismissive attitudes about memory difficulties as being "just a normal part of aging" and "just come back when it is bad enough to put you on medication."

Well, let me tell you something. I don't like that dismissive attitude and I know that doing nothing is not a way to outsmart dementia. There actually are things that you can do to improve your brain health and decrease the chances of dementia. These are mistakes that I have reported during CBS, ABC, NBC, and FOX TV news talk interviews that you can watch at http://www.TheRedwoodClinic.com/media-kit. And if you don't know why you should take the time and effort to avoid dementia and Alzheimer's starting right now, you can go to my website http://www.outsmartingdementia.org that has vignettes of experiences people have had with dementia and Alzheimer's and you can watch such movies as "Still Alice."

What is Dementia and What are Some Types of Dementia?

Dementia is a general term for loss of memory and other mental abilities severe enough to interfere with daily life. It is caused by physical changes in the brain. A list of different types of dementia includes the following: mild cognitive impairment, posterior cortical atrophy, Down syndrome, traumatic brain injury, Alzheimer's, vascular, dementia with Lewy bodies, mixed dementia, Parkinson's disease, frontotemporal dementia, Creutzfeldt-Jakob disease, normal pressure hydrocephalus, Huntington's disease, and Wernicke-Korsakoff syndrome (associated often with alcoholism).

Memory loss that disrupts daily life may be a symptom of Alzheimer's or another dementia. Alzheimer's is a brain disease that causes a slow decline in memory, thinking and reasoning skills. It causes a degeneration of functioning.

As I have reported during TV news interviews on CBS, ABC, NBC FOX and CW around the country -- and completely based on scientific and medical studies -- there are three things that you should avoid to help prevent from getting Alzheimer's and dementia. If you do not avoid these and correct the issues, your health will suffer in other areas as well. My purpose with this book is to help you avoid Alzheimer's and successfully keep your brain safe, sharp, and sexy into the future.

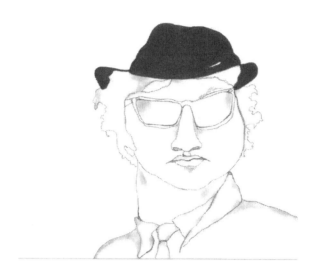

The "John Belushi"

The first one I call "The John Belushi." John was a large man and a comedian. It is great to laugh. It is essential to laugh in life for so many reasons. On the other hand, obesity is no laughing matter from a health perspective.

So, with respect to Alzheimer's and dementia, the first thing to avoid is obesity. Obesity is an extreme form of being overweight. According to the Kaiser Family Medical Foundation, obesity and overweight conditions lower brain function. In fact, the more fat you have on your body, the smaller your brain becomes! You might be thinking "I know many people who are overweight or obese who are really smart." But, in the long run obesity is a liability for risk factors associated with brain degeneration and damage, like having a stroke and developing crusty brain syndrome. Obesity is a risk factor for many other conditions, but those are not the focus of this book.

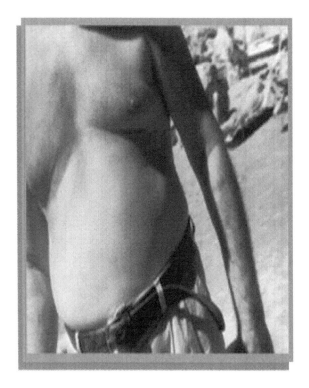

Would you like to know if you are overweight or obese? You probably have a good idea already, but to get specifics on your body composition, read on.

There are several ways to determine whether you are in a healthier weight range for your personal situation, or whether you are overweight or obese. There are 5 major ways to determine this from measurements. You can measure your hip to waist ratio with a measuring tape, you can use a buoyancy tank, you can use bioimpedance analysis, you can use skin calipers, and you can use BMI. The most common methods is using a BMI (Body Mass Index) Chart. You line up your height and weight (no cheating on the figures!) and then determine your BMI (body mass index) from the chart. A 19-24 BMI is considered in the healthier range. A 25-29 is overweight and 30 or higher is obese. I like to use the bioimpedance analysis in the clinic as it is accurate and takes into account and individuals personal circumstances.

A full 80% of Americans are overweight or obese, putting them at greater risk of developing Alzheimer's or dementia. This increased risk was found to be true in a scientific study done by Kaiser Permanente researchers in 2013. It bears repeating, it has also been discovered that THE MORE (Visceral) FAT YOU HAVE, THE SMALLER YOUR BRAIN becomes. Visceral fat means fat accumulating around your organs as opposed to fat under your skin. Visceral fat accumulates around your liver, heart, intestines, as opposed to fat located under your skin, which is called cutaneous fat. Are you setting yourself up for dementia and small-brain syndrome due to too much fat? If you are, take this seriously! You need to address this now -- there are healthy options and programs to help you improve your body composition mentioned at the end of this chapter. My training in several effective systems to help Improve body composition gives me a great way to help others reduce their brain risk factors through programs at The Redwood Clinic. These include the use of medical foods, detoxification, and exercise.

Did I tell you that the Kaiser Family Foundation also did a study, based on real patients over 20 years that concluded that the risk of dementia is increased with the greater amount of visceral fat on your body? (No, I did not forget that I just wrote that! The competent brain needs to hear something repeated at least 3 times to start to get it to stick – I am not simply being redundant.)

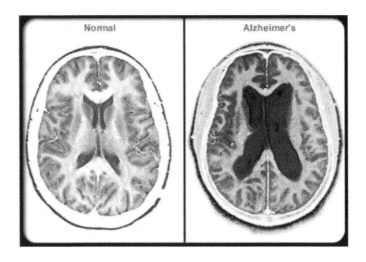

The breakdown of the brain -- and decreased nerve density and power associated with Alzheimer's -- is shown in comparison to a normal brain. You can see more "black" areas on the right, indicating that the nerves have degenerated and thus the brain tissue has shrunken. Cerebrospinal fluid, contained within the meningeal membranes. Fills the space up like a swimming pool liner filled with more water as the swimming pool gets bigger. These normal spaces in the brain are called ventricles.

21

BODY MASS INDEX (BMI)

The higher your BMI, the higher your health risk

EMI ➤	19	20	21	22	23	24	25	26	27	28	29	30	31	32	33	34	35	36	37	38	39	40	41	42	43	44
		◀	HEALTHY	▶			◀	OVERWEIGHT	▶			◀						OBESE								▶
Height/Weight												weight (lbs)														
4'10" (58")	91	96	100	105	110	115	119	124	129	134	138	143	148	153	158	162	167	172	177	181	186	191	196	201	205	210
4'11" (59")	96	99	104	109	114	119	124	128	133	138	143	148	152	158	163	168	173	178	183	188	193	198	203	208	212	217
5'0" (60")	97	102	107	112	118	123	128	133	138	143	148	153	158	163	168	174	179	184	189	194	199	204	209	215	220	225
5'1" (61")	100	106	111	116	122	127	132	137	143	148	153	158	164	169	174	180	185	190	195	201	206	211	217	222	227	232
5'2" (62")	104	109	115	120	126	131	136	142	147	153	158	164	169	175	180	186	191	196	202	207	213	218	224	229	235	240
5'3" (63")	107	113	118	124	130	135	141	146	152	158	163	169	175	180	186	191	197	203	208	214	220	225	231	237	242	248
5'4" (64")	110	116	122	128	134	140	145	151	157	163	169	174	180	186	192	197	204	209	215	221	227	232	238	244	250	256
5'5" (65")	114	120	126	132	138	144	150	156	162	168	174	180	186	192	198	204	210	216	222	228	234	240	246	252	258	264
5'6" (66")	118	124	130	136	142	148	155	161	167	173	179	186	192	198	204	210	216	223	229	235	241	247	253	260	266	272
5'7" (67")	121	127	134	140	146	153	159	166	172	178	185	191	198	204	211	217	223	230	236	242	249	255	261	268	274	280
5'8" (68")	125	131	138	144	151	158	164	171	177	184	190	197	203	210	216	223	230	236	243	249	256	262	269	276	282	289
5'9" (69")	128	135	142	149	155	162	169	176	182	189	196	203	209	216	223	230	236	243	250	257	263	270	277	284	291	297
5'10" (70")	132	139	146	153	160	167	174	181	188	195	202	209	216	222	229	236	243	250	257	264	271	278	285	292	299	306
5'11" (71")	136	143	150	157	165	172	179	186	193	200	208	215	222	229	236	243	250	257	265	272	279	286	293	301	308	315
6'0" (72")	140	147	154	162	169	177	184	191	199	206	213	221	228	235	242	250	258	265	272	279	287	294	302	309	316	324
6'1" (73")	144	151	159	166	174	182	189	197	204	212	219	227	235	242	250	257	265	272	280	288	295	302	310	318	325	333
6'2" (74")	148	155	163	171	179	186	194	202	210	218	225	233	241	249	256	264	272	280	287	295	303	311	319	326	334	342
6'3" (75")	152	160	168	176	184	192	200	208	216	224	232	240	248	256	264	272	279	287	295	303	311	319	327	335	343	351
6'4" (76")	156	164	172	180	189	197	205	213	221	230	238	246	254	263	271	279	287	295	304	312	320	328	336	344	353	361

Chart adapted from The National Institutes for Health Web site Body Mass Index Table page.

This is one of many examples of a BMI – Body Mass Index – Chart. All BMI charts have 3 components. Height, weight, and BMI. The height is always either listed in the left side column or across the top row. Body weight (in pounds or kilograms) and BMI are either in the left column or top row OR in the inside of the chart. In this chart the weight is in the body of the chart and the BMI is listed across the top. This chart also shows the associations of the BMI numbers and the classifications: Healthy, Overweight, and OBESE across the top of the chart under the BMI. The higher your BMI, the higher your health risk.

Using this chart, to find YOUR BMI, find your height along the left hand column. Go to the RIGHT across the row that corresponds to your height until you get to your weight (don't cheat!). Then go UP that column of your weight (corresponding to your height) to find your BMI. Is it in the Healthy, Overweight, or OBESE category? If you are overweight or obese you have some serious work to do (unless you are a top athlete and your muscle mass is so high that your weight tips you over into a higher BMI. Evander Hollifield is one such example of a highly muscular athlete who has a high BMI but low fat mass.) If you are not a top athlete, it is time to get started of be more persistent in finding a program that works for you.

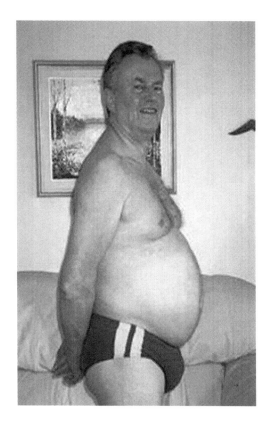

The look of Obesity in a Speedo Swimsuit

Addressing overweight and obesity, especially with visceral body fat is important for your health and the health and wellbeing of those around you. For further information about effective programs to address this go to http://www.TheRedwoodClinic.com/healthy-body-composition.

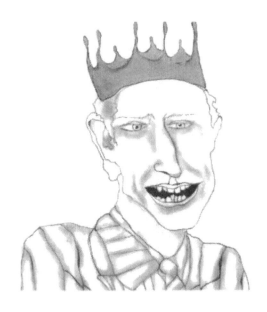

Illustration of Prince Charles on Late Late Show

The "Prince Charles"

The second thing to avoid is what I call "The Prince Charles." Craig Ferguson used to make fun of Prince Charles on the Late Late Show. He portrayed Prince Charles as having very bad teeth. The importance of taking care of your teeth and gums is an area of health that is well known but often neglected. The fact that it can also effect the brain is a discovery that I have been sharing with the public on television since spring 2014.

Inflammation or infection of the gums or mouth not only effects the mouth, teeth and sinuses, but also has significant impact on the overall health of the body and brain. Infections or chronic inflammation of the mouth and gums can result in inflammatory influences in the sinuses and the brain. That can cause a breakdown in the brain's defense mechanisms. This is damage to the blood-brain barrier and can lead to "leaky brain syndrome." Leaky brain syndrome is a situation where the brain is exposed to allergens, toxins, and inflammatory reactions that it is normally protected from. All of these cause irritation to the brain and nerves and can lead to a breakdown of the brain and spinal cord.

So what should you do? Brush and floss your teeth, get regular dental care, and cut down on acidic and sugar-rich foods to prevent teeth cavities as well as "brain cavities" that are seen on the MRIs of patients with Alzheimer's! I am not saying that the "brain cavities" on MRIs come from bad dental care, but it could be contributory. And poor dental hygiene can lead to halitosis, and bad breath is not sexy. See the later Chapter 10 in this book on this topic!

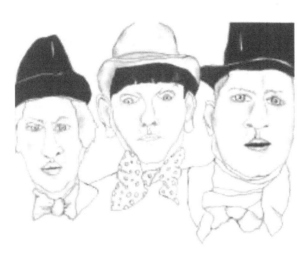

The Three Stooges and Cumulative Traumas from Head Injury

The "Three Stooges"

The third thing to avoid is what I call "The Three Stooges." Curly, Larry, and Mo are the Three Stooges, comedians I grew up watching on Saturday morning TV as many of you did as well. Their slap-stick comedy is classic. It portrays the common injuries that happen to people throughout their day-to-day living – falling down, jarring the head and neck, direct blows to the head, running into doors, walls, windows, etc. We all have had these experiences in life if we have lived long enough. And, as a child I seem to recall mimicking those Three Stooges antics with my sisters much to the chagrin of our parents.

I personally think that there is something funny about self-deprecating humor -- allowing us humans to laugh at ourselves and the mistakes we make. Laughing at our mistakes can help take the sting out of them. (At the same time, laughing at others' mistakes and misfortunes can also be a tendency that some of us can fall into easily if not careful.)

Having these injuries as a matter of simply living is inevitable. However, the Three Stooges had these types of injuries, as wells as getting "slapped up aside the head," over and over in very short period of time. These were repetitive injuries. In the Three Stooges series these antics were considered to be funny and nothing to be taken seriously. They were just stooges after all.

But in real life, repetitive blows to the head should be taken seriously. Just laughing about such injuries is TRIVIALIZING them. Why would that be the case? Because these injuries cause damage to various parts of the head and neck as well as other parts of the body. In particular, because these injuries cause damage to the meninges, the meninges should be examined periodically and taken care of therapeutically. You may be wondering, "What are the meninges?"

What are the Meninges?

The meninges, for those who don't know or have forgotten, are three, thin, "plastic-wrap-like" membranes that surround and protect the brain and spinal cord. (As a side note, the repair of meningeal compression and torqueing may be achieved by means of NRCT (Neurologic Relief Center TechniqueTM), a practice I have been trained in and use with great effect with numerous patients with seizures, tremors, peripheral neuropathy, tingling, chronic pain, and brain fog, to mention a few of the conditions and symptoms that have responded to this system.)

Further information on NRCT, the meninges, and patients who I have helped can be accessed online at www.theredwoodclinic.com/nrct-faqs.

Example of Effects of Helping Undo Meningeal Compression

For example, one 26 year old woman and student came into me because of a severe brain fog and fatigue that caused her to drop out of college. After 8 weeks of treatment she was able to return to a normal life, full of hope and the ability to again engage in student life and family activities. We saved her life and the lives of those patient and loving people who had been her caregivers. If we hadn't been able to help, she probably would have continued to face exhaustion, unable to work or study, costing her a valuable life, using her partner's life simply as a caretaker, and costing hundreds of thousands, if not millions, of dollars in medical costs over her lifetime as her life and health broke down. What a great feeling that was for me and my staff, being able to help a woman regain her life. Fortunately, we get to do this frequently - help to turn the life around of people in very difficult situations who were not helped sufficiently because the meningeal compression component was not discovered or corrected by other caregivers.

How the meninges are related to head injuries are explained in a news appearance I made in Las Vegas. Watch it at http://www.TheRedwoodClinic.com/media-kit

These chronic, cumulative injuries can also effect other tissue structures in the body, such as the muscles, tendons, ligaments, and bones of the head, neck and shoulders as well. These small injuries, if not corrected, accumulate over time. Just like creases and lines on the face that can become furrows with repetition over time.

While the body has an innate healing ability, repeated injuries can cause a buildup of scar tissue, inflammatory responses, and dysfunctional muscle-use patterns that become more difficult to change. Sometimes they become permanent changes that are so disruptive to other tissue structures that damage results, and that change causes pain and breakdown of the body. For example, some tall people would have the habit of banging their head on a door frame because door frames (in the U.S.) are standardized for a person between 72-75 inches tall. A person who is even 75 inches tall, 6' 3" (six feet three inches) tall would constantly hit their forehead on a door frame. Thus, they will learn to avoid hitting their head by ducking. Over time they tend to slouch when walking because of an avoidance of door frames. I see this all the time in my practice over 30 years. Slouching caused by door frame avoidance behavior leads to damage of many other parts of the body, including damaging breathing!

Unfortunately, early evaluation and treatment is not occurring to the degree necessary to ward off dementia and the symptoms of "normal aging." The medical system, based on insurance billing and payments in 5 minute intervals and cursory symptom oriented office visits is not taking these vital issues of your brain health seriously. Only private evaluations are really taking the time to look at and address these important issues seriously.

The "Gibbs"

I might have also called it "The Gibbs" in honor of Jethro Gibbs, the head of the NCSI (Naval Crime Scene Investigators). "NCSI" is a very popular CBS television program -- if you didn't hear of it before. Agent Jethro Gibbs, the boss, has a habit of hitting his "probies" (the new Agents who are on probation) up the side of the head to tell them to wake up and get it together. While it is a memorable character behavior that fits well into a very popular TV series, that type of blow to the head is the exact type of trauma that can lead to meningeal compression and torqueing that we NRCT clinicians find can lead to neurological damage and symptoms.

What are other examples of traumas that can lead to meningeal compression and torqueing that we NRCT clinicians find can lead to neurological damage and symptoms? These traumas include repeated athletic injuries to the head due to impacts on the football, hockey, and soccer fields. They can be related to war -- concussion injuries due to explosions in the battlefield. They can also be from automobiles -- whiplashes occurring in car injuries. All of these traumas are what I am talking about. They are sometimes called traumatic brain injuries (TBI). Or when it is a repeated injury, this is called chronic traumatic encephalopathy (CTE). Encephalopathy means a disease process or lesion of the head. Each of these head and neck traumas may seem minor at the time. However, as they accumulate, the impact is amplified on the brain and nervous system.

Bicycle Accident of My Tai Chi Chuan Student - Friend

A single traumatic injury to the head can be devastating. In the 1970's I taught Tai Chi Chuan classes at Earlham College as part of the physical education program. This class was quite popular. I learned a particular form of Tai Chi Chuan my freshman year of college from Don Weed who had studied with Da Liu in New York City. I had the great honor, privilege, and fun to teach many of my student colleagues this amazing exercise/martial art/meditation/health form. A dear college friend of mine who I taught Tai Chi Chuan to had a bicycle accident during the years I was away in Japan and travelling across Asia. When I returned to live in Philadelphia for several years I took an acupuncture program in Columbia, Maryland. I used to commute to the program and I was honored to be able to stay at his mother's home with him in Baltimore during the years of study. Michael had had a bicycle injury while going downhill and it severely affected his ability to walk and speak. He remembered only part of it; I recall that his foot got caught in the pedal as his brakes locked up and threw him over his handlebars, his head twisted to the side as his head braked his body across the asphalt a long distance down that steep slope. People stopped to help him and to get an ambulance. Needless to say, his road to recovery was long and arduous, with so much loving support from his mother, brother, and others around him. He still remained the incredible person I knew from Earlham College in spite of his injury. He had great will power bolstered by the love of those around him. If he had worn a helmet his injuries might not have been so severe.

This illustrates that TBI is not something to make light of though. Chris Borland, Christopher Reeves, Payton Manning, Mohammed Ali, and George Clooney all suffered head injuries that had significant impacts, changing their careers. So this type of event is not uncommon.

Seeking Care Early-On for Head Injuries is Key

Seeking care is VITAL to undo the cumulative traumas these minor (or major) whiplash and impact injuries impose on the brain. It is also VITAL to prevent irreversible damage to the nervous system tissues that keep us functioning. While you might think that everything is fine because you have no noticeable symptoms, function can be affected. Symptoms are the

29

last evidence that there is a breakdown in your body's function, When function is effected the body has already undergone some degeneration. The more malfunction continues the more likely disease is going to occur. The foundation of symptoms is malfunction and disease – symptoms are the last things to develop and they (symptoms) tell you that you have neglected to address the process of degeneration and loss of function. Watch my video explanation of the functional medicine approach to understanding how your symptoms develop from a decreasing of function due to stagnation and deficiencies of blood, oxygen, nutrients, hormones and control messages. Stagnation decreases functioning. Stagnation and most health problems come from stress, traumas, and toxicity. http://www.TheRedwoodClinic.com/symptoms-as-loss-of-function.

A stroke is a great example of this process. It may be a process that takes a long time to develop but the suddenness of the symptoms, paralysis, loss of speech, drooping face, some combination of the above or worse, makes us think that the symptoms are the problem. The symptoms are the result, not the cause. So, the build-up of small traumas, one on top of the other is the cause of what is to come. Chronic problems, cumulative injuries, lead to chronic traumatic encephalopathy, also known as CTE.

The seriousness of CTE in the sports field is now more widely recognized. Chronic Traumatic Encephalopathy has even lead to depression and suicide in several famous sports figures. Preventing this condition, CTE, has led to campaigns and new legislation that now requires helmet for particular sports when they didn't exist before. Also, the style of coaching particular sports has changed. This has occurred in many states. This is a counter-trend to the mentality of trivializing these injuries as personified by the Three Stooges.

Nevertheless, early evaluation and treatment is not occurring to the degree necessary to ward off the damaging effects of CTE, dementia and the symptoms of "normal aging." The medical system, based on insurance billing, payments in 5-minute intervals, and cursory, symptom-oriented office visits is not taking these vital issues of your brain health seriously. In my clinical experience and from what my patients tell me, only private evaluations are really taking the time to look at and address these important issues seriously.

So it is important to start evaluating yourself and loved ones to see if the early signs of brain degeneration are occurring. This is not to mean that coming up with a poor result on a survey definitely means that you have brain degeneration or that your brain is shrinking. However, it does mean that there is something going on that needs to be looked at more in depth by a professional who knows what to look for in a more comprehensive way. These surveys will help you better understand if you should get qualified medical help.

On the following pages are some surveys specific to what we are talking about.

Complete these **SURVEYS to see if any of your injuries may be influencing your brain.**

EMOTIONS

Enter the appropriate number - 0, 1, 2, or 3 - with 0 as least/never and 3 as most/always

___Mood Swings

___Anxiety, fear, or nervousness

___Anger, irritability

___Depression

___Sense of despair

___Uncaring or disinterested

___TOTAL   If your total is 6 or more I suggest that you get evaluated more in depth. See Chapter 12

ENERGY/ACTIVITY

Enter the appropriate number - 0, 1, 2, or 3 - with 0 as least/never and 3 as most/always

___Fatigue or sluggishness

___Hyperactivity

___Restless

___Insomnia

___Startled awake at night

___TOTAL

If your total is 6 or more I suggest that you get evaluated more in depth. See Chapter 12

MIND

Enter the appropriate number - 0, 1, 2, or 3 - with 0 as least/never and 3 as most/always

___Poor Memory

___Confusion

___Poor Concentration

___Poor Coordination

___Difficulty making decisions

___Stuttering, Stammering

___Slurred speech

___Learning disabilities

___TOTAL

If your total is 6 or more I suggest that you get evaluated more in depth. See Chapter 12

CHAPTER 4: DR. JAY'S "B.R.A.I.N.S." FORMULA

To help people remember some key elements to maintaining a healthy brain (and memory), I have come up with my B.R.A.I.N.S. FORMULA. Each letter of the word "BRAINS" represents something that you have to think about and address in your life to successfully stay safe, sharp, alert, sexy, productive, and have an engaged life with family and friends.

B stands for Blood Circulation.

R stands for Remove toxins

A stands for Avoid Sugar

I stands for Inflammation

N stands for Names

S stands for Sexy

In the following chapters I will explore and expand upon these 6 elements in my BRAINS formula. I chose these 6 elements because I feel that they will have the biggest positive impact on reversing this epidemic of dementia. There are many other elements to health and brain protection that can have an impact. The Alzheimer's Association and brain researchers at UCLA and elsewhere have stated that a multifaceted approach is necessary to address Alzheimer's. I wholly agree with this and do not think that there is a "silver bullet" discovery or drug that will change this trajectory.

But in coming up with my BRAINS acronym I had many approaches and elements to choose from, so let me mention a few others that I will not discuss in great detail, but that have influence nevertheless on dementia.

B: B-vitamins are very important in brain and nerve health. Some, like B12, are not processed efficiently by some people and this then needs to be addressed with the proper form of B12 added to the diets of these people, L-5- methyl tetrahydrofolate, available at our online store (http://www.theredwoodclinic.metagenics.com). Blood sugar is a key B which is included in the "A" letter chapter. Balance in life is important -- this is both the balance needed to walk, run and sit, but also a balance in all parts of one's life. And Boredom at work and elsewhere can be a negative influence on the brain.

R: Rest and relaxation/fun is important. Hanging out in one's "man cave," "woman cave," vacationing, doing recreation that reduces stress responses. Stress is a big killer of brain function and is discussed in greater detail in "Super Brain: Maximize Your Brain Health for a Better Life." Remember to Brush and floss your teeth properly daily.

I: Immune system dysregulation causing "leaky brain syndrome" and meningeal leakage as well are mentioned in this book elsewhere. Food coloring attaching to tissues like the tongue can lead to immune attack and brain irritation and breakdown. Insulin is also a key factor in brain health.

N: Neurologic Relief Center Technique for meningeal compression and torqueing. Discussed elsewhere in this book.

S: Staying Safe and Sharp. This book is mostly about staying safe firstly, and sharp thereafter.

CHAPTER 5: "B" STANDS FOR BLOOD CIRCULATION

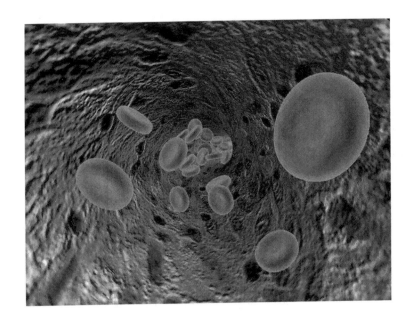

Red Blood Cells Carrying Oxygen in the Blood Stream

What happens when blood and oxygen are cut off from your brain?

Our brain, like all parts of the body, requires blood and oxygen circulation to function properly. A lack of blood or oxygen to any part of the brain for even a short time will result in malfunction and even permanent damage. A stroke is an example of this. This is why it is very important to take steps to keep your blood vessels open and filled with sufficient amounts of oxygen and high quality blood. How can we do that?

Acupuncture, NRCT (Neurologic Relief Center Technique), yoga, Tai Chi, other exercises, relaxation and meditation techniques, and certain natural supplements and herbs are necessary components of your health care routine to support healthy blood circulation as well as to undo negative influences of things like whiplash and "Gibbsian" blows to the side of the head.

My work as an acupuncturist, traditional naturopath, and NRCT practitioner has helped hundreds of patients with blood and oxygen deficiency and stagnation issues damaging their bodies and brains. Restoring proper function is a satisfying aspect of my work in helping others optimize their health. If you haven't done so already, watch the video explanation on how function is related to symptoms, stress, trauma, and toxicity at http://www.TheRedwoodClinic.com/symptoms-as-loss-of-function

One thing many other practitioners overlook is the role of oxygenation in health. Anemia, low blood iron and decreased hemoglobin are a source of numerous symptoms a person might ascribe to other causes. When oxygen deficiency is not addressed, not only do symptoms persist and get worse, but the whole body's function is diminished. Anemia is more common in women than men due to the loss of blood during the menstrual cycle. So keep in mind that oxygen deficiency due to anemia can be a key concept for women and men who are having memory issues. Oxygen is needed by the brain to function properly, and circulation of blood to the brain through both the carotid and vertebral arteries are necessary for proper levels of nutrients and oxygen getting to the brain. The meninges are the "wet suit" gate keepers of the flow of blood and oxygen to the brain from the circulatory system. This "wet suit" function is also called the "blood-brain barrier."

After the oxygen and nutrients get to the brain and nerve cells, mitochondria, the power houses of the cells, have to have the proper nutrients to produce the energy. Supplements such as mitochondrial resuscitate assist in that function.

Massage, shiatsu, chiropractic, osteopathic manipulation and various forms of exercise and meditation can increase the flow of blood to the brain by relaxing the muscles of the shoulders, and neck as well. Blood to the brain is transported from the heart through the carotid and vertebral arteries. The carotid artery, which we all know about in the front of the neck, carries about 60%, the vertebral (lesser known) carries the other 40%. Tension in the neck and shoulder muscles causes decreased flow of blood through the vertebral artery. This was a discovery by Dr. Yoshiaki Omura during his research as a cardiologist. While there is redundancy built into our body to allow for damage and decreased flow, getting full flow of blood to the brain is really a key to healthy function. Thus, doing the above methods is a very important part of what any health care system should include and they are approaches I use in my own blend of help to support my own health and the health of patients.

Answer the questions in the following SURVEY to see if BLOOD CIRCULATION may be an issue for you:

BLOOD CIRCULATION

Enter the appropriate number - 0, 1, 2, or 3 - with 0 as least/never and 3 as most/always

___Low brain endurance for focus and concentration.

___Cold hands and feet

___Must exercise or drink coffee to improve brain function

___Poor nail health

___Fungal growth on toenails

___Must wear socks at night

___Nail beds are white instead of pink

___Tip of your nose is cold

TOTAL___ If your total is 6 or more I suggest that you get evaluated more in depth. See Chapter 12

CHAPTER 6: "R" STANDS FOR REMOVE TOXINS

Toxins have always existed in our environment. Humans have learned which things make them sick and poison them, and which things make them healthy and strong. Sometimes it has been obvious; other times it has taken decades to really finally figure out that things we thought were health-producing are actually damaging to our bodies and brains.

Compared to 100 years ago, our environment is now filled with many more potential toxins. According to experts worldwide, there are more than 100,000 (one hundred thousand!) new chemicals in the environment that never existed before on this earth. That is because we humans created them to make things like cars, airplanes, computers, and cell phones. On the other hand, very few have actually been tested for their toxic or physical effects on the body, so their safety is unknown. These chemicals are man-made, artificial, not natural to the Earth. Think about it. Is your cell phone made of wood, plants, or parts of animals? While the chips are made of modified sand (silica), you just can't put together a cell phone by going out into the woods and collecting things from nature. So these 100,000 new chemicals are not natural and our bodies have never had to encounter them in the past. These chemicals are all new things for the immune system, cells, and tissues to figure out when the touch the body and if they get into the body. My chart below illustrates this extreme change over the past 100 years.

Many substances in the environment are neurotoxic. This means that they damage nerves and the brain which is composed of nerve cells. Well known neurotoxins include pesticides, volatile organic solvents, mercury, lead, aluminum, and cadmium. Clearing these chemicals and heavy metals out of our bodies is undeniably an important thing to do to reduce chances of memory loss, decreased brain ability and intelligence, tremors, Parkinson's, and other nasty degenerative conditions.

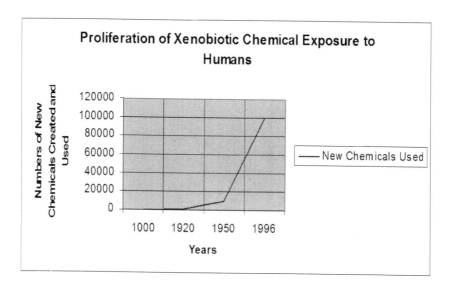

Proliferation of Xenobiotic Chemical Exposure to Humans

Other chemical toxins must be removed from our body to prevent nerve damage as well. Carbon tetrachloride, asbestos, pesticides, herbicides, and various plastics, to mention only a very few, are neurotoxic and cannot stay in our bodies without our expecting damage to be done. A long list of chemicals that can be found in drinking water and their effects can be found at http://www.TheRedwoodClinic.com/toxins-in-water A Multipure carbon block filter is tested to remove these substances to 99% by independent lab testing, so I recommend that all of my patients and people I care about to use this system for all their drinking and cooking water needs. http://www.multipureusa.com/redwoodclinic

There are certain primary organs and systems in our body that clear out toxins. Supporting our liver, gall bladder, bowels, kidney and spleen is a necessary and key memory care action to prevent chemical toxic buildup from killing us. Further information on this process is available in lectures you may access through a special membership site http://www.TheRedwoodClinic.com/clearing-toxins

To stay as healthy as possible you must remove toxins that are in your body and avoid putting more toxins into your body. Our bodies are more than 72% water. Removing toxins from the body is done primarily by making them more water soluble so that we can pee them out, poop them out, spit them out, sweat them out, and cry them out. The liver makes them more water soluble by a several step process. However, we want to prevent them from getting them into the body via water, food, air and skin contact. Thus, preventing toxins from getting into the body through our drinking water is a reason why everyone should use a water filtration system. Again, I highly recommend the Multipure system. http://www.multipureusa.com/redwoodclinic. The Multipure systems are easy to use, independently tested by Underwriters Laboratory testing, easy to install, and have decades of reliability. I have used them in my home and at clinics since 1983.

You can also get information in video format online at the above website as well as by signing up for my video series on toxicity, water purification, and heavy metal toxicity testing at http://www.TheRedwoodClinic.com/Removing-Toxicity

How do we know if our body is clearing out heavy metals or other damaging chemicals properly and effectively? We can use modern laboratory testing that either detects the presence of the toxins, the presence of antibodies to the toxins, testing of your body's neurologic response to toxins, or testing the detoxification processes in your body and how competently they are removing the toxins. The pH of your saliva can be an initial simple test of toxic build-up in your body. That is one of the screening tests that we do onsite in our company wellness programs that corporations hire us to do for their wellness programs. Testing can be fairly generalized and less expensive and then be very specific and more expensive. But where health is concerned, what you spend to deal with toxicity in your body pays off big benefits in the future. Just think about the poisoning of Victor Yeshenko with a drop of DDT in his martini during the Ukrainian elections many years ago and the impact this can have on your life is more real.

But suffice it to say that there are tests we can use to help elucidate toxicity and dysfunction of your liver, kidneys, and other routes of detoxification as well as foci of toxicity in your body. With that information we are able to support your body's ability to remove some of the toxic influences that will lead to damage of the brain and can lead to dementia. A detailed program for your particular situation is the best approach, but assuming that you do have toxicity in your body is a good bet. General supplementation that helps with detoxification support can be found online at http://www.theredwoodclinic.metagenics.com and other non-online sources we use to help patients.

Complete the <u>SURVEY below to see if you may have symptoms of toxicity</u>:

SYMPTOMS OF TOXICITY

Enter the appropriate number - 0, 1, 2, or 3 - with 0 as least/never and 3 as most/always

___Acne and unhealthy skin

___Excessive hair loss

___Overall sense of bloating

___Bodily swelling for no reason

___Hormonal imbalances

___Weight gain

___Poor Bowel Function

___Excessively foul-smelling sweat

___ TOTAL   If your total is 6 or more I suggest that you get evaluated more in depth. See Chapter 12

SURVEY of RISK OF EXPOSURE

Enter the corresponding number

0=Never 1=Rarely 2=Monthly 3=Weekly 4=Daily

___How often are strong chemicals used in your home? (disinfectants, bleaches, oven and drain cleaners, furniture polish, floor wax, window cleaners, etc.)

___How often are pesticides used in your home?

___How often do you have your home treated for insects?

___How often are you exposed to dust, overstuffed furniture, tobacco smoke, mothballs, incense, or varnish in your home or office?

___How often are you exposed to nail polish, perfume, hairspray, or other cosmetics?

___How often are you exposed to diesel fumes, exhaust fumes, or gasoline fumes?

___TOTAL   If your total is 8 or more I suggest that you get evaluated more in depth. See Chapter 12

SURVEY of ENVIRONMENTAL FACTORS

Enter the Corresponding number

0=NO 1=Mild Change 2=Moderate Change 3=Drastic Change

___Have you noticed any negative change in your health since you moved into your home or apartment?

___Have you noticed any change in your health since you started your new job?

Answer Yes or No (Yes = 4)

___Do you have a water purification system in your home?

___Do you have any indoor pets?

___Do you have an air purification system in your home?

___Are you a dentist, painter, farm worker, or construction worker?

___TOTAL   If your total is 8 or more I suggest that you get evaluated more in depth. See Chapter 12

CHAPTER 7: "A" STANDS FOR AVOID SUGAR

Your body produces energy from sugar and your brain requires sugar to operate. However, that sugar (glucose) is produced internally and so we usually don't need that form of sugar in our diet directly. In other words, rarely do you need to put simple sugars in concentrated forms into your mouths to feed your body. (In a hospital setting a glucose intravenous drip line is used, but that is not an everyday condition for most people). That type of eating causes an inflammation-inducing condition in your body, setting you up for pre-diabetic tendencies at a low level, repeatedly, over and over again. Eventually that up and down sugar exposure causes deterioration of the body's function and inflammatory reactions in the brain. Brain inflammation then can lead to deterioration of memory and other functions. You have heard of diabetes. Alzheimer's is classified as Type III diabetes. In other words, Alzheimer's is sugar-related. That is why it is being called Type III diabetes. High blood sugar also induces release of insulin and leptin, an appetite control substance.

Nutrition Tip: Starting the morning out with protein in your breakfast meal is known medically to buffer the shocks of sugar in the system and to reduce sugar craving. There are many other ways to help buffer the shocks of sugar on your system and to reduce sugar craving that take into account your individual metabolic needs. A hair mineral analysis may be able to help discern the best way for you, as a unique individual, to approach this. More information on hair mineral analysis is found at http://www.TheRedwoodClinic.com/hair-mineral-analysis.

Is it any wonder that there are problems with sugar metabolism when consumption of refined sugar has sky-rocketed? The next chart shows this rise.

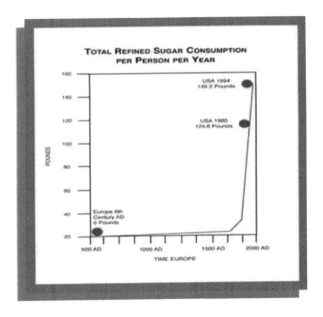

This is a chart showing the unbelievable increase

in the consumption of refined sugar in the U.S.

Dot 1 (far left): Europe 6th century AD

Dot 2 (middle): USA 1980

Dot 3 (far right): USA 1994

Soft drink consumption is one major source of this.

Our stress-balancing program has helped many overweight people lose weight as a positive side effect. Our weight loss / healthy body composition program also reduces stress as a positive side effect. Go to our membership site to view videos on stress and on weight loss programs.

Hypoglycemia and hyperglycemia are two conditions related to blood sugar balance and imbalance. <u>Fill out the surveys below</u> to see if you might have either or both of these.

HYPOGLYCEMIA AND HYPERGLYCEMIA

Enter the appropriate number - 0, 1, 2, or 3 - with 0 as least/never and 3 as most/always

____Crave sweets during the day

____Irritable if meals are missed

____Depend on coffee to keep going/get started

____Get light-headed if meals are missed

____Eating relieves fatigue

____Feel shaky, jittery, or have tremors

____Agitated, easily upset, nervous

____Poor memory /forgetful

____Blurred vision

____Fatigue after meals

____Eating sweets does not relieve cravings for

sugar

___Must have sweets after meals

___Waist girth is equal to or larger than hip girth

__Frequent urination

__Increased thirst and appetite

__Difficulty losing weight

__TOTAL

If your total is 8 or more I suggest that you get evaluated more in depth. See Chapter 12

CHAPTER 8: "I" STANDS FOR INFLAMMATION

Current research tells us that inflammation is one of the most significant factors related to decreased body function in general and brain degeneration specifically. Diabetes is a condition of dysregulated blood sugar levels. Dysregulation means a loss of regulation and decreased control over the crucial sugar balancing system of the body. Diabetes is also an inflammatory condition.

Long term diabetic patients have cognitive (thinking) disorders and memory difficulties. I have personally experienced what diabetes can do to the memories (and other parts of the body) in both clinical settings and personal experiences with relatives. My much-admired and loved role-model Uncle Russ was a surgeon. In his later years he had advanced diabetes, leading to amputation of limbs and coma-like periods of awakeness in a nursing home setting. Also, my Aunt Dottie (my father's brother's wife) had advanced stage diabetes that led to periods of memory loss, inability to recognize relatives and children who came to visit, and episodes of coma-like states. Diabetes is not the only inflammatory condition that can occur in the body. But, any broadly significant inflammation, including that in the intestines, can significantly impact the brain in a negative way. Thus, reducing diabetic tendencies and reducing inflammatory responses like gluten and other food sensitivities will help reduce the inflammatory factors that cause brain degeneration.

For further information on how inflammation influences the functioning or your body, go to our membership sites and watch videos on gluten, inflammation, diabetes, SIBO (small intestine bacterial overgrowth), how to save your brain, etc.

Some of the supplements and medical foods that can help you address this inflammatory condition include ClearVite, UltraInflamX, UltraMeal360, a cinnamon product (MetaglycemX), all available online at http://www.TheRedwoodClinic.metagenics.com. Other supplements designed specifically for brain inflammation, poor blood circulation, and gluten sensitivity can be obtained by calling The Redwood Clinic to create a personalized program. It is best to have a comprehensive functional medicine evaluation before starting to take these supplements and medical foods.

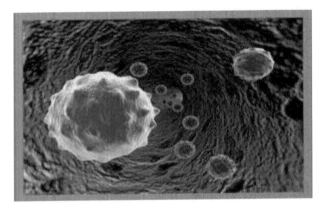

White Blood Cells Circulating in the Blood Stream are an Important Part of Your Immunity

Your level of inflammation and areas of inflammation in your body are what we begin to discern in our consultation program. I help you know what areas must be addressed to reduce inflammation and memory damage. See the resources page here for details. This process includes testing for stress responses, toxicity and traumas as well.

Take the <u>SURVEY below related to stress and inflammation</u>.

STRESS AND INFLAMMATION

Enter the appropriate number - 0, 1, 2, or 3 -, with 0 as least/never and 3 as most/always

___Cannot stay asleep

___Crave salt

___Slow starter in morning

___Afternoon fatigue

___Dizziness when standing up quickly

___Afternoon headaches

___Headaches with exertion or stress

___Weak nails

___Cannot fall asleep

___Perspire easily

___Under a high amount of stress

___Weight gain when under stress

___Wake up tired even after 6 or more hours of sleep

___Excessive perspiration or perspiration with little or no activity

___TOTAL   If your total is 7 or more I suggest that you get evaluated more in depth. See Chapter 12

CHAPTER 9: "N" STANDS FOR NAMES

The way that we remember other people's names is by association. We associate a person's name (a sound and a series of written words or symbols) with a face, a voice sound, a feeling, a series of experiences, smells, emotions, and other things. This is how memories of names are created. These different types of associations involve different parts of the brain. Sounds in one area, images in another, smells in even another, and emotions &feelings diffusely in many areas of the brain. Thus, practicing remembering names of people you have met helps your brain to access and use different parts of the brain. This improves brain flexibility of nerves (neuroplasticity) and helps to integrate different parts of the brain related to memory power.

Initial signs of dementia include forgetting names of pets. After you do our basic online brain assessment, we can fine tune areas of your brain that are showing signs of malfunction or non-optimal functioning and then create plans to potentially recover function if the condition is not too severe.

Complete the survey online to see if you are starting to have some indications or signs of memory loss.

"N" is Also for Nutrition

There is a lot of truth in the saying "You are what you eat." Targeted nutritional supplementation may also help you stay sharp and clear-headed. Extensive research demonstrates the brain-supportive benefits of huperzine A (found in Chinese club moss) and a special proline-rich polypeptide (PRP) complex from colostrum. Huperzine A positively affects the neurotransmitter acetylcholine that is involved in important cognitive processes like memory. And in a clinical trial, 50% of those supplementing with the PRP complex showed stabilization in overall score for memory, language, orientation, and simple tasks. The other 50% showed significant improvement compared to placebo. This PRP complex may also help support other functions related to healthy brain aging, such as protecting the integrity of brain cells and fighting excess oxidative stress that can damage cells throughout the body. This is a particular nutritional regimen that is available through The Redwood Clinic following the comprehensive consultation. Call for more information   +1-510-849-1176.

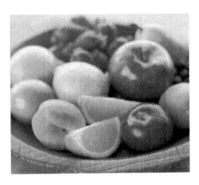

You can sign up for our natural health newsletter and subscribe to our blog. Like us on Facebook (/RedwoodClinic). Call today to set up a consultation to learn more about healthy brain aging—especially if you're experiencing signs of age-related cognitive decline. Because, "How much is your brain worth to you?"

Check out your brain health with an initial online survey you can do by registering your copy of this e-book and your copy of the paper version.

Get an analysis of your overall health and functioning by signing up and filling it out online. We will send you an analysis of your Health Appraisal Questionnaire.

Eating the right foods is important. Avoiding foods that you are immunologically sensitive to is equally important. If you don't have an obvious and severe reaction to a food you still might be sensitive to certain ones. To reduce inflammation that can cause brain degeneration knowing what foods you are sensitive to is important. Testing for food allergies can take various forms. Elimination diets and reintroduction with notation of reactions. Eliminating gluten. Eliminating night shades. Eliminating the most typically allergenic foods. IgA, IgE, IgM and IgG antibody testing. RAST (skin) test. White blood cell sensitivity testing. The most appropriate test depends upon your circumstances. Our membership site has more information about these tests. For a personalized evaluation call The Redwood Clinic for an appointment.

CHAPTER 10: "S" IS FOR SEXY!?

You might be asking, "What does SEXY have to do with dementia? What *is* the relationship between the brain and sex, the brain and sexual attraction, memory and sexual attraction?"

Well, the adage that "what makes for good sex is what is between your ears" certainly applies to both men and women. While gonads are an important hormonal driving force in sexual activity, experts agree that good sex is more about what is between your ears than what's between your legs. Sex hormones are primarily produced in the ovaries and testes, but hormones related to things such as sex drive, interest, and energy levels are also produced in the brain and other parts of the body.

The brain is an emotional organ and emotions (and motion) are definitely related to the brain and memory.

We are not just talking about the fact that your brain stem, the locus of survival actions and emotions – like procreation and replication of the species – is literally located between your ears. Other, higher order brain functions exist there as well. Intelligence, wit, humor, playfulness, thoughtful skill, communication, other-orientation-before-self, big picture and details, planning – these are all major keys to a healthy, happy, and satisfying sex and intimacy life for both women and men.

We don't need scientific studies to let us know that sexual activity is good for all parts of the brain. (Although there is a lot of scientific study that shows and details just that!) The high emotional content of sexual activity engages many parts and aspects of the brain – imagination, memories, colors, sounds, emotions, taste, smell, touch – and the cortex, cerebellum, mid-brain, brain stem, spinal cord, peripheral nerves, and autonomic nervous system. (If you don't understand these terms, learn more in Super

Brain: Maximize Your Brain Health for a Better Life.) So the survival brain and the "new brain" are involved in a coordinated fashion.

A number of chemicals in the brain are associated with memory and other functions and emotions. Having sufficient amounts of these neurotransmitters and feel-good chemicals, naturally produced by the brain due to various stimulations and activities, is important for a healthy brain and a happy life. Losing memory capabilities, dementia, is a definite killer of deeply satisfying sexual activity. Dementia can rob a person (who has dementia) of many of the positive personality traits that made them attractive to others. Dementia also can rob a person of their ability to remember how to do all the things they did for their partner(s) that helped to satisfy them sexually, mentally, emotionally, physically, and spiritually.

An imaginative mind can be sexy. A wandering mind can be a bane to sexy and intimacy. Thus, it is valuable, and enhancing to the sexual experience, to practice being in the moment, focused on what is going on right now. Not being able to shift gears in the brain, from imagination and memories to being in the now can dampen the moments of deep intimacy. A degenerating brain has difficulty focusing and having executive control. So, avoiding dementia is definitely related to being and staying sexy.

What are some the chemicals in the brain related to feeling good? Well, some women will say that female orgasms are literally addictive because when a woman comes, her brain is flooded with TONS of endorphins and other pleasure-inducing chemicals like dopamine and oxytocin... The exact same chemicals that get released in the brain when someone takes a drug like cocaine or heroin!

Women's brains are wired this way because women are actually much more likely to conceive a child when they reach climax. Experts suggest that these pleasure chemicals are a woman's body's reward system to keep them having sex with men who can make them come. In reality, women don't need a man to help them reach climax, and there are many ways to reach climax.

Dopamine is a neurotransmitter that is one key chemical related to brain function and memory. It is also lacking in people with Parkinson's, one of the forms of dementia.

Endorphins are the feel-good chemicals the brain produces also after a long run. They are an antistress chemical, and stress is bad for memory. Acupuncture is also known to increase endorphins.

Orgasms for men also flood his body with feel-good chemicals that incidentally are also needed for the brain to remember and function in full capacity.

So not only does preventing dementia help you to keep your brain safe, sharp, and sexy into the future, having sex can help you stave off dementia due to the whole action that it has on many parts of your brain and the chemicals that flood your brain during intimacy, whether reaching orgasm or not.

If you are interested in improving your orgasm-providing skills, suggested sources are available on our membership site.

CHAPTER 11: Summary

This book is an outgrowth of a series of news interviews I have made on ABC, CBS, NBC, CW, and FOX promoting my book called "Super Brain: Maximize Your Brain Health for a Better Life" and sharing my message that there are things you can do to help avoid Alzheimer's. This book amplifies the points that I bullet pointed on television. These included the 3 Things to Avoid to Prevent Alzheimer's and Dr. Jay's B.R.A.I.N.S. Formula. We have gone into more detail to explain why I emphasized those to the television audience and we are providing you with resources to take charge of your brain health. Why should you act now?

"Procrastination is like a credit card:
It's lots of fun until you get the bill."
–Christopher Parker

"The most common cause of

bankruptcies in the US is due to

medical bills that cannot be paid.

More than 80% of medical costs go to

chronic illness and end-stage medical

and hospital care." Act NOW to

prevent a bigger cost for you and your

family in the future.

CHAPTER 12: RESOURCES

Throughout this book we have given you various websites to go to get further information or the chance to get surveys analyzed. A more comprehensive evaluation is possible by calling The Redwood Clinic and setting up an appointment. There is also an online store where you can purchase supplements manufactured by a very reputable and reliable company. These supplements are referred to in this book.

ABOUT THE AUTHOR, JAY SORDEAN, LAC, OMD, QME, CTN

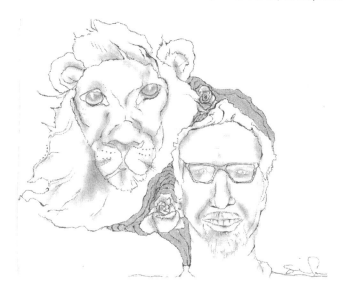

Thousands of patients have benefited by the evaluation and treatments using acupuncture, herbs, naturopathic supplements, shiatsu massage, NRCT, weight loss programs, detoxification programs, and other modalities with Dr. Jay Sordean. In order to promote his mission to prevent 1 million cases of dementia and Alzheimer's, best-selling author and clinician Dr. Jay has appeared on televisions stations around the U.S., including ABC, CBS, NBC, FOX, and CW. Dr. Jay has lectured to diverse audiences on keys to preserving their brains and memory. He is available to TV appearances and as a speaker on brain health, improving memory, and company wellness programs that address these issues.

Training and Credentials

Dr. John R. "Dr. Jay" Sordean uses his medical experience—as a licensed acupuncturist (L.Ac.), Oriental Medical Doctor (O.M.D.), Certified Traditional Naturopath (C.T.N.), Qualified Medical Evaluator (Q.M.E.), homeopath, and herbalist—to promote an understanding of good health for culturally diverse communities.

Dr. Sordean has treated an extensive range of health issues, and specializes in the brain, pediatrics, immunology, orthopedic and neurological acupuncture, and herbology. He has been certified as a Diplomate of Acupuncture by the National Certification Commission for Acupuncture and Oriental Medicine and the National Board of Acupuncture Orthopedics.

In 2005, he achieved Medical Provider certification in the First Line Therapy program, which leads patients to optimal health and body composition through balanced eating, exercise, stress reduction, appropriate testing (toxicity, body mass), and nutritional supplements.

In 2009, Dr. Sordean completed training in the Neurologic Relief Center Technique to treat fibromyalgia, chronic pain, migraine headaches, Parkinson's, TMJ, MS, and rheumatoid arthritis.

Less than one percent of California and national licensed acupuncturists have achieved this level of advanced training.

Focus on Oriental Medicine

Fluent in Japanese, Dr. Sordean offers his patients techniques and treatments rare among Western doctors. He began his study of Oriental Medicine with Tai Qi Chuan and Shiatsu and immersed himself in Japanese culture while at Earlham College, a Quaker school. Dr.Sordean's formal training in acupuncture and herbology began on a 1973 trip to Japan, and continued in China (Taiwan, Hong Kong); his homeopathic training included clinical study in Calcutta, India. He later earned Practitioner of Classical Homeopathy status from the Dynamis School of Advanced

Homeopathic Studies, in Canada.

Public Service

Dr. Sordean has been active in Northern California community affairs since his move to Berkeley over 30 years ago. He has been a member of the Berkeley, Emeryville, Albany and Richmond chambers of commerce and has given educational talks to Rotary, Kiwanis, hospitals, police, senior centers, and other service groups. He served on the Board of the California Acupuncture Association. He serves on the board of the Berkeley Sakai Association (a sister-city non-profit), H.A.A.R.T., and the People's Life Fund.

Patient Satisfaction

Dr. Sordean's clients cite his sensitivity and expertise in resolving their individual needs— treatment for acute pain, chronic disease, work or personal injury—or promoting lifelong good health and disease prevention. Patients also value his open communication with their primary- care physicians and his advocacy of a holistic and preventative approach to health. See http:// www.theredwoodclinic.com for testimonials and other conditions we treat effectively.

Recommended by the Author

Alzheimer's Association: A source about Alzheimer's and local and national resources and events related to Alzheimer's and dementia for caregivers. www.alz.org

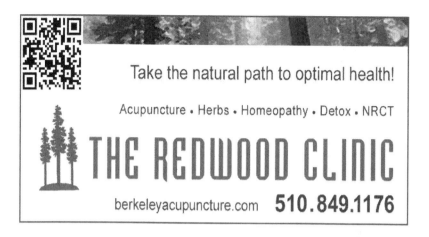
The Redwood Clinic

3021 Telegraph Avenue, Suite C, Berkeley, CA 94705: A natural medicine clinic with expertise in evaluation and natural treatment of neurological and brain health issues from a wholistic perspective.

CALL TODAY: +1-510-849-1176

For a free brief online brain assessment

& to sign-up for a Free Video Education Course on "How to Protect Your Brain"

www.TheRedwoodClinic.com/Removing-toxicity

NOTES:

NOTES:

24414889R10046

Made in the USA
San Bernardino, CA
23 September 2015